~~[name]~~,

So proud to call you friends!
May God open all the doors
as you Trust His timing.

1 Cor 1:8-10

Broken &
BLESSED

by Jim Risner

Risner Press, LLC

ISBN: 979-8-218-22739-5   979-8-218-22740-1 EPUB

jim@jimrisner.com

Broken & Blessed
Risner Press, LLC.

A CIP record for this book is available from the Library of Congress Cataloging-in-Publication Data

Dedicated To

Barb: my first (only) wife, and ministry partner.

Our Children: Brett and Debra, Bethany and Jeff, Jeremy and Darci, Jennifer and Paul.

Our Grandkids: Cam, Will, Maddie and Kai, Kate, Franky J, Robbie, Cali, Carson, Chase.

Our Great Grandkids: ...

Table of Contents

Broken &
BLESSED

Introduction
God' Surrounding Love

My name is James David Risner. You can call me Jim. Now that we're friends, I'll tell you why I wrote these poems. I've wrestled with depression since I was in high school (1970). Yes. I'm old.

I've come to understand what the triggers are, but it's taken a lifetime to accept and accommodate them.

When I sat in the psychiatrist's office for the first time, he asked if I'd *ever been happy.* I wasn't sure how to answer. Several months prior to this visit, I'd had one of my worst episodes.

I've always found, writing a song or a poem alleviated my pain. So, during a six-month period, I wrote. It's been several years since that time. My friends encouraged me to make my poems available.

So, dear reader, if these words bring any comfort, I'm honored. More importantly, *thank God for His surrounding love.*

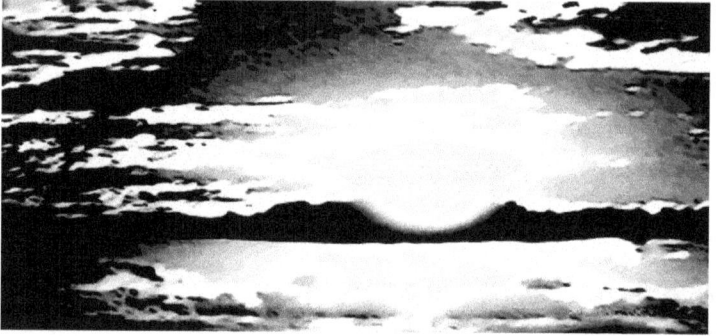

The LORD is a refuge for the oppressed, a stronghold in times of trouble.

Psalms 9:9,10

1
I Will Praise You

I will praise you Lord for you are good.
Even in the midst of trouble you are righteous.
The enemy of my soul, the enemy of my life is no match for you.

You hold me in your hand.
Your peace is my pillow.
Your joy my blanket in the cold of night.

Your greatness cannot be contained in the universe.
Your words are living sounds.
Each word you speak brings life or death.

Engulf me in your presence.
Let your Spirit come and transform me.
May each fiber of my being be secured in your love.

I will praise you and only you.
Troubles are no match for your grace and mercy.
I will praise you and only you.

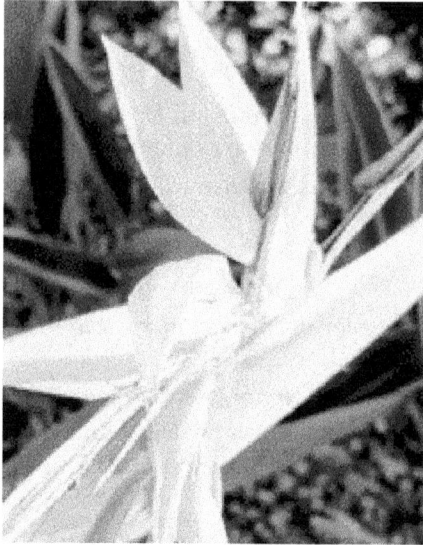

Create in me a pure heart, O God, and renew a steadfast spirit within me.
Psalms 51:10

2
Have Mercy

O Lord, my sin is ever before me;
have mercy on me.
That which I know is right to do
slips through my grasp like holding onto the wind.
That which I know is wrong
clings to me like a bur on a horse's mane.
Surround me by your presence.
Seal my mind from wondering destructive paths.
Have mercy on me.
Capture my heart so it will be true to you
and not its evil intent.
Have mercy on me.
Let my eyes focus on you the Almighty.
Let my ears hear the whisper of your Spirit.
Have mercy on me.
Let my wondering cease
that I may journey with you,
My Friend, My Savior, My God.

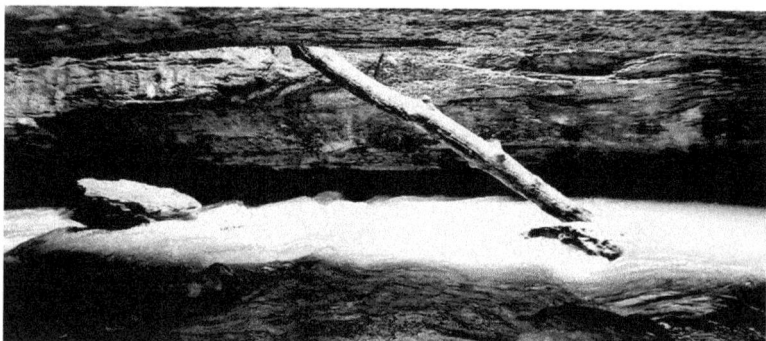

We were under great pressure, far beyond our ability to endure, so that we despaired of life itself ... Indeed, we felt we had received the sentence of death.

2 Corinthians 1:8,9

3
Depressed But Not Defeated

O Lord, look on me with pity.
The habits of my mind have destroyed me.
My heart and mind have conspired.
The destruction of my soul is their delight.

But you are greater than my mind.
You created my heart.
O Lord, rescue me from myself.
Let me stand in the light of you love.

Defeat the darkness of depression.
Make me whole by your presence.
Give me strength to fight.
Give me strength to stand still.

Uphold me with your righteousness.
Overwhelm me with your joy.
Rescue me with your peace.
And I will continually praise your name.

'Why, my soul,
are you downcast?
Why so disturbed
within me?
Put your hope in God,
for I will yet praise him,
my Savior and my God.

Psalm 42:11

4
Why Not Me

Why not me, Lord, why not me.
Others are promoted; am I so unfaithful?
Others seem to catch all the breaks, why not me?
Others seem to have joyful lives, why not me?

Circumstances are not the issue.
Earthly promotion is not the goal.
You are such a gracious God - why me.
You continue to bless when there is no reason.

Your love is greater than my faults.
Your presence surrounds me when I don't deserve it.
You are unfailing in your care for your children.
Why me Lord, why me.

O Lord. It is all about You!

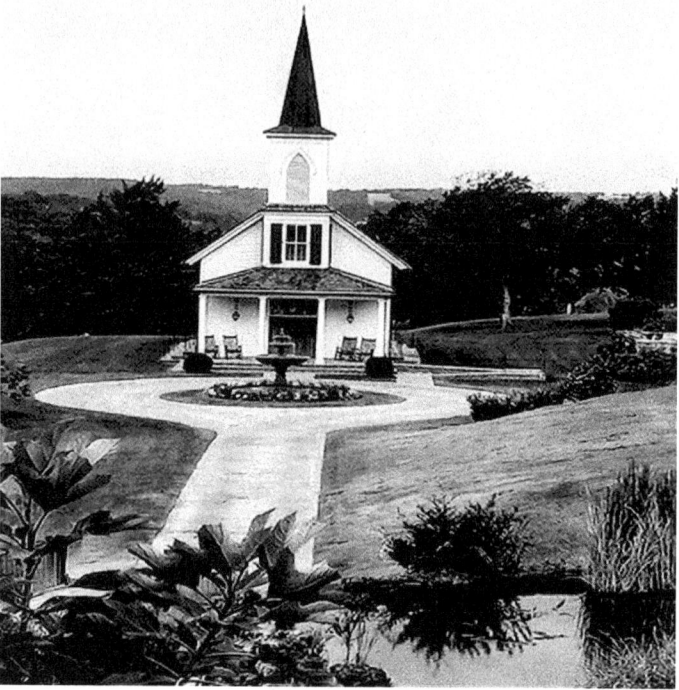

... If we are faithless, he remains faithful, for he cannot disown himself.

2 Timothy 2:13

5
You Are Faithful

O Lord, I am living in the land of famine.
I didn't see the signs?
I ignored the signs?
I refused to see the signs?
O Lord, I have no foresight
and my hindsight has grown fuzzy.

I am at your mercy.
You alone know the motivations of my heart.
But, I have never refused to go where you have directed.
I have been as generous as I know how to be.
When I have seen a person in need of a job I have helped them.
I have carried some even after I should have let them go.
I have given of my time and resources to invest in your kingdom.

You do not refuse anyone forgiveness.
Those who repent stand inside your arms of protection and
mercy. You love to provide for your children.
O lord, forgive my selfish heart, I repent of my trusting in self.
I am your child, bless me Father or I will die in this land of
famine.

You are faithful, and I will bless your name.
You are faithful, and I will count your blessings.
You are faithful, I will accept your crushing and your discipline.
You are faithful, do not hide your face from me.
You are faithful, I will put my hope in you.
You are faithful, I will wait for the rain and
the manna of your blessing.

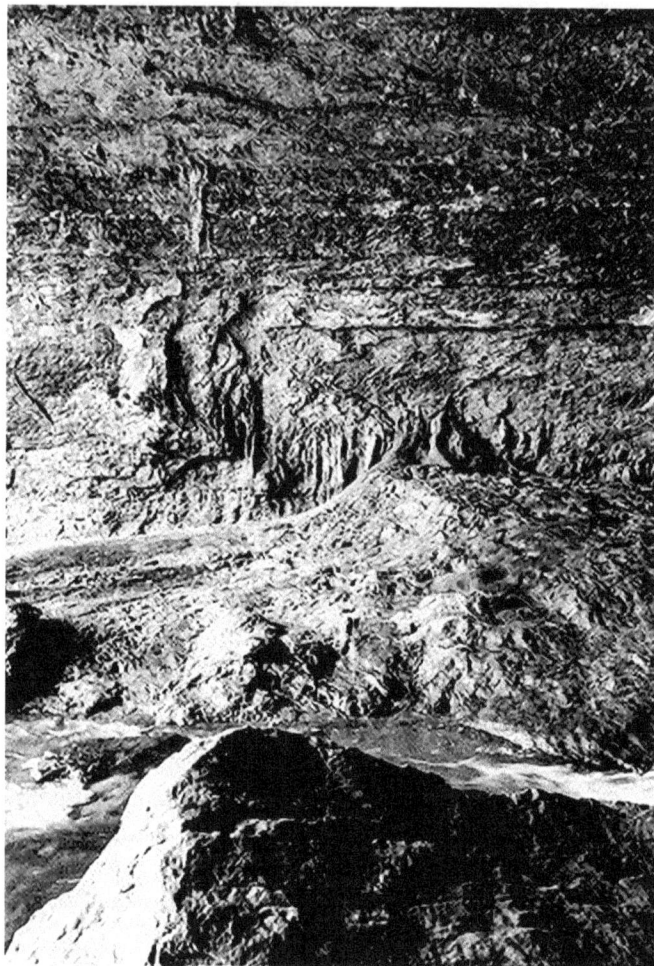

LORD my God, I take refuge in
you; save and deliver me from all
who pursue me ...

Psalms 7:16

6
Rescue Me

O Lord, rescue me from this fiery pit.
destroy the enemy of my soul.
bring clarity to my mind.
If rescue circumvents knowing you better,
leave me here.

You alone know how much I can bear.
I commit my spirit into your hands.
But I need your peace, I need your joy.

Overcome my melancholy.
Overrule my emotions.

Let me trust in your unfailing kindness.
Let me rest in arms of mercy.
Let your grace wash over me
like the oil of anointing.
Above all else,
I want to know you.

In the midst of turmoil and chaos,
I will worship you.
I will sing your praise.
I will walk with you.
My Savior, Defender, and Friend.

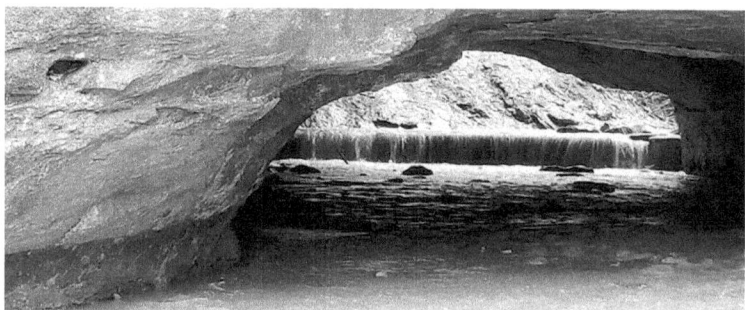

Answer me when I call to you, my righteous God. Give me relief from my distress; have mercy on me and hear my prayer.

Psalms 4:1

7
Hear My Prayer

O Lord, teach me to fear you.
Help me cross the line from fearing circumstance and people
to fearing only you.

Cause my heart to be strengthened by your presence.
Cause my mind to be disciplined by your wisdom.
Cause my will to grasp the peace at bowing at your throne.

May your Spirit come, hear my request.
Your Word is true.
Your perfect love drives away fear.

Come now and loosen the chains of fear.
Destroy the shackles that have held me bound.
Burn the walls of the prison that have held me fast.

You do not refuse the cry of your children.
Hear my prayer, O Lord, and answer me.
I will be careful to always praise your name for delivering me.

LORD, hear my prayer, listen to my cry for mercy; in your faithfulness and righteousness come to my relief.

Psalms 143:1

8
Ruin

O Lord, I am facing ruin.
Are you turning away from me?
My soul withers away like a flower in the desert.
Will those who watch, gloat over my failure?
Will they say, "God can't be trusted?"
Not for my sake, but for theirs,
Answer my prayers, hear my groaning.
Do not delay.
My demise is close at hand.

Speak the word and I am free.
Let my heart rejoice in your comfort.
Let my ears be deaf to those who would scoff.
May your Spirit intercede on my behalf.
May your angels do battle against the enemy.
Hear my prayer - I wait for you.
You do all things well.
You see beyond the moment.
I will rest in you.

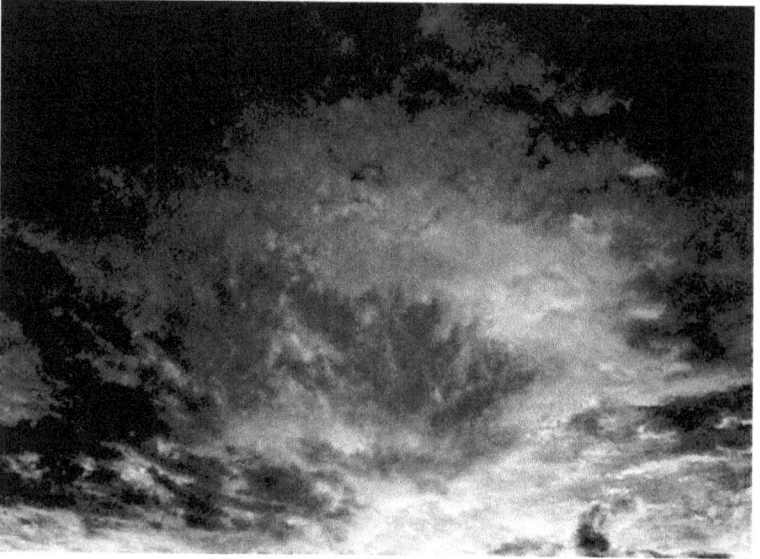

I call on the LORD in my
distress, and he answers me.

Psalms 120:1

9
Distressed but Determined

O Lord, in my distress I cry out to you.
I know in my heart you have not abandoned me.
But my eyes still focus on the circumstance.
You allow nothing into our lives that will destroy us.
Your desire is to make us stronger,
to rely on you more.

O Lord, I have done your work all my life.
But the work be damned.
If I don't know you better, the work gains me nothing.
Others may benefit, to you be the glory.

Lord, I have to be honest,
I don't like the pain of growing up.
But like the butterfly, I will continue to struggle
so I may soar with you.

From the ends of the earth I call
to you, I call as my heart grows
faint; lead me to the rock that is
higher than I.

Psalms 61:2

10
Stuck In-Between

O Lord, I am stuck In-between,
I am no longer the idealistic youth.
And yet, I do not feel like a wise old man.

Lord, I am stuck in-between.
All the things I thought I knew...I don't.
The things I need to know, I have no grasp of.

I no longer know how you are leading me.
I no longer seem to hear as I should.
My sight is growing dim.

All I have is in jeopardy.
All that I thought you gifted me to do gone.
I am broken, bruised, and battered.

I have tried to be your servant.
I am angry at you.
I am undone.

You are not stuck in-between.
You are constant from beginning to end.
In-between is where faith is tested, and trust is lived.

Whatever my sin, you have forgiven.
Your mercy and grace are my consolation.
I ask not for rescue, but sustenance to see me through.

Let me learn more of your companionship.
Let your peace overshadow me.
I will Worship You.

Living in the land of blessing,
Or in-between...
I Will Worship You.

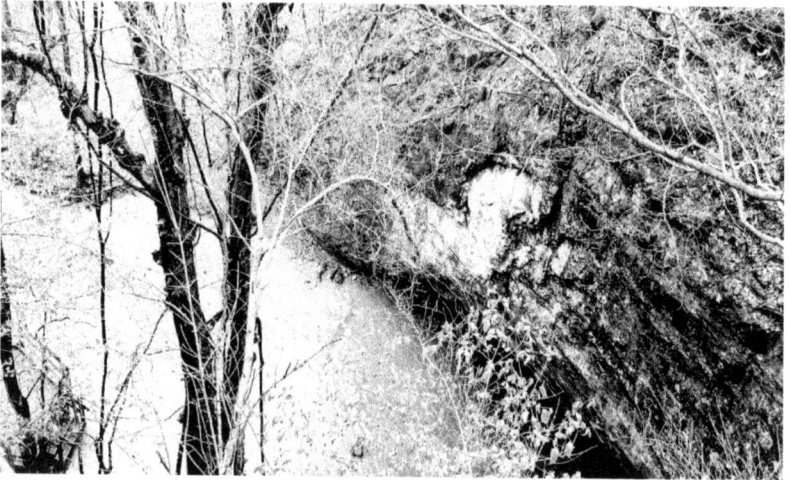

But I trust in your unfailing love;
my heart rejoices in your
salvation. I will sing the LORD's
praise, for he has been
good to me.

Psalms 13:5,6

11
Standing in the Flood

*O Lord, some days getting to you
is like walking through a monsoon flood.
I try with all my might, but can't get any closer.
All that is around me pushes back and interferes.*

*Lord, look on me; Father, I cry out to you.
Help your faltering child.
Your presence is the only safe place.
Your presence is my only protection.*

*Fill me with your strength to stand against the flood.
Fill me with your Spirit so our connection is secure.
Fill me with faith to see beyond the present onslaught.
Fill me with joy so I may love life.*

*I will praise your name.
I will shout of your greatness.
I will sing of your goodness.
I trust in you.*

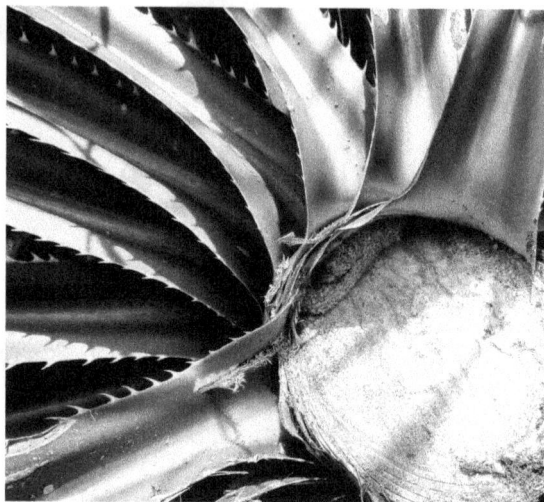

Do not let your heart envy
sinners, but always be zealous
for the fear of the LORD.

Psalms 23:17

12

Jealousy and Envy

O, Lord, why do jealousy and envy rage against me.
These twins of destruction pierce my soul.
They whisper in my ear,
"Others are successful, when will you?"
"Others are promoted, why not you?"
"Others have opportunity, why not you?"

Lord, rebuke these interlopers.
Send your Spirit to seal me in your presence.
I willingly place my body, mind, and spirit in your keeping.
You create my paths.
You direct my steps.

Lord, I refuse their companionship.
I will no longer listen to their siren call.
Forgive me for allowing them access to my heart.
I reject their enticement.

Success is living in obedience to your Word.
Promotion is walking in your presence.
Opportunity is loving others.

Companionship with you is the only worthy pursuit.
Walking in your Spirit is the greatest prize.
You are God and I am Yours!

But I trust in you, LORD; I say,
"You are my God."

Psalms 13:14

13
Trust in You

O Lord, I declare my trust in you!
You are faithful.
You do all things well.
You delight in your children.
Their success makes you proud!

Teach me to walk in peaceful obedience.
Your design for me is greater than anything I can imagine.
Your provision is more than adequate.
Your presence is life.

O Lord I declare my trust in you.
When war is declared against me
I will stand in your armor.
When I am powerless against the foe
I will hide in you.

When My feet have taken me down the wayward path
You lovingly guide me back to your side.
When I fall into the pit
you rescue me.

When I have been blinded by the glitter of stuff
You gently heal my sight.
When I have been deafened by the siren call of success
You whisper my name and I hear again.

When my hands have created idols
You cleanse my hands so I may lift them in worship to you.
When I am puffed up by others compliments
You kindly remind me where the gift comes from.

When my mind has conceived grand plans for myself You
show me yours and I am humbled by your trust in me.
When my heart declares independence
You graciously remind me only in you am I at my best.

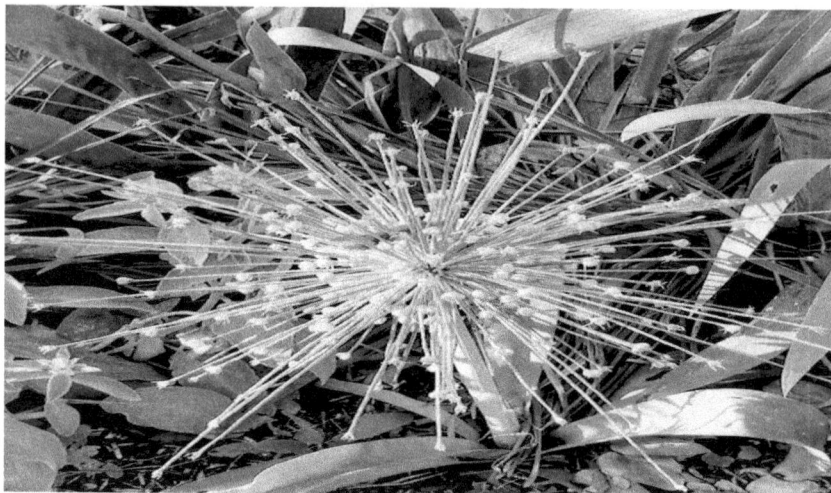

The LORD is my strength and my
shield; my heart trusts in him,
and he helps me.
My heart leaps for joy, and
with my song I praise him.

Psalms 28:7

14
I Don't Want to be Happy

O Lord, everything in this world
tells me to seek happiness:
Seek it in what I have,
Seek it in what I do,
Use others to my own happy ends,
Find my happy place.

Happiness is not a destination.
Happiness is a drug.
It is frantically bought and sold daily.
It is a temporary fix for a permanent problem.
Happiness rises and falls with the circumstances.

Lord, I don't want to be happy.
I want to be joyful.
You are the source of joy.
You are joy.
Only relationship with you brings joy.
May your Spirit well up within me.
May your joy overflow from your presence within.
I choose Joy.

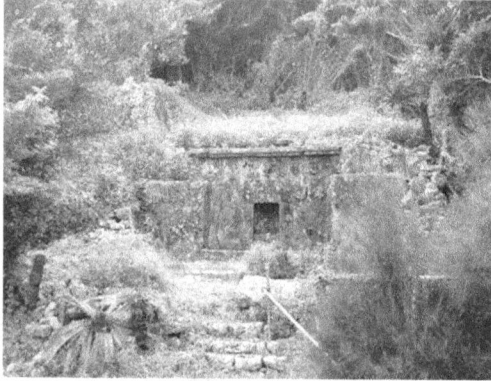

Keep me safe, my God, for in you I take refuge.

Pslams 16:1

15
My Hiding Place

O Lord, you are my hiding place,
You are the refuge of my soul.
When I am at odds with myself
and the world around me,
You open your arms and draw me in.

When I have grown weary from the struggle
You are my rest.
Help me remember the battle is yours.
It is not in confrontation
but in relaxing in your presence.

Whatever the result of each circumstance
- you are God.
You can be trusted.
Teach me to be satisfied with you and you
alone.

You are my Refuge, my Strength, my Rest.

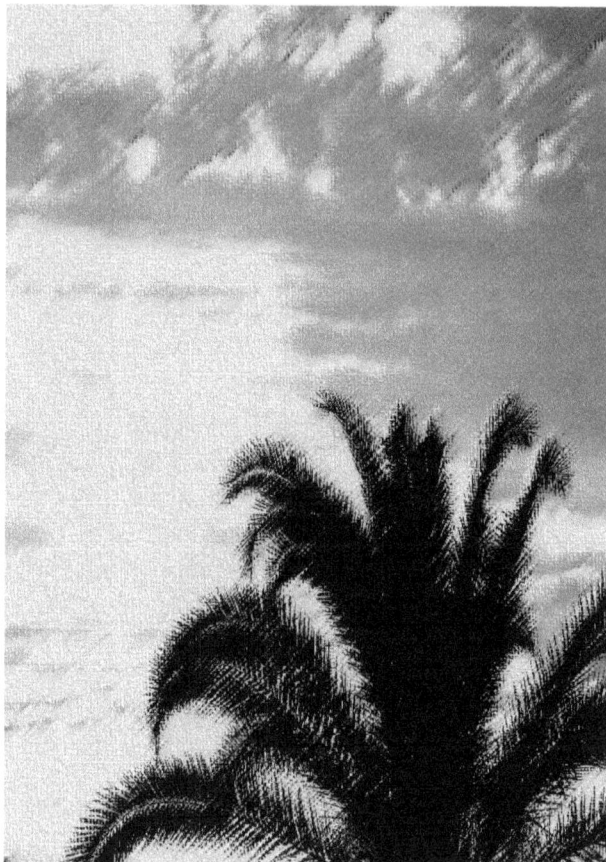

In the morning, LORD, you hear
my voice; in the morning I lay my
requests before you and
wait expectantly.

Psalms 5:3

16
Morning Praise

O Lord, in the morning I will praise your name.
Your grace and mercy are my constant companions.
Your Spirit goes before me and prepares my day.
I will bless your name.

My heart will sing your praise throughout the day.
Whether good or ill befall me, my song will rise to you.
My words and actions declare your glory
to all who hear and see me.

When day ends I will rest in your peace.
For you and only you bring satisfaction.
You alone restore my body, mind and soul.
Even as my eyes close in sleep my heart rejoices in you.

But blessed is the one who trusts in the LORD, whose confidence is in him.

Jeremiah 17:7

17
Confidence

O Lord, you are my confidence.
In you I will trust.
When others curse your name
I will worship you.
When others question your reality
I will believe in you.

When trials block my path
You will show me a way.
When temptation trips me
You lift me up and lead the way.
When Pride detours me
You gently lead me back.

You have declared your power and might.
You have declared there is no God but you.
You have declared your Word is everlasting.
You have declared your care for your children.
You have declared your Spirit is with those who love you.
I declare - you are my confidence.

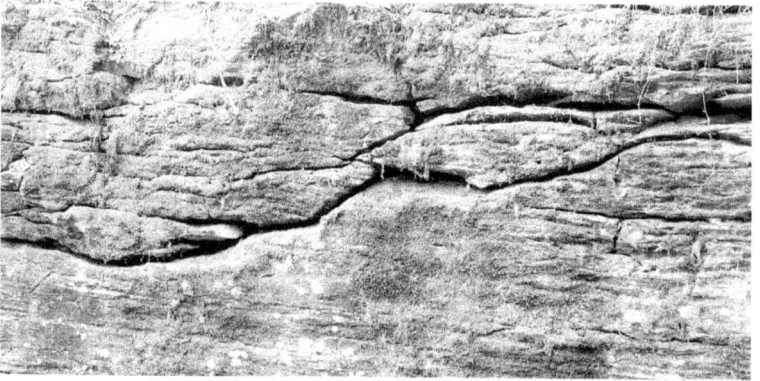

Be strong and courageous. Do not
be afraid; do not
be discouraged, for the LORD
your God will be with you
wherever you go.

Joshua 1:9

18
Courage

O Lord, give me courage to stay the course.
My all you have designed for me come to pass.
When I wonder, hedge me in.
When mistakes of the past begin to march through my mind,
rain on the parade.

When I begin to judge myself by earthly criteria,
remind me I live in your kingdom.
Show me continually what kingdom success is.
It is not in breadth of position, power, and prestige,
but in depth of relationship with you.

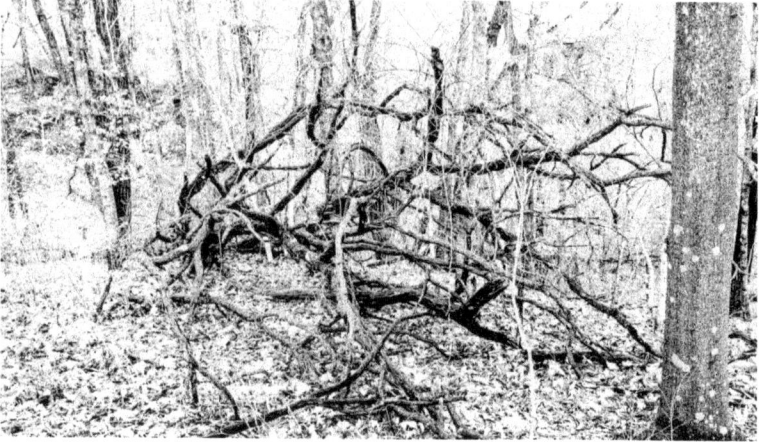

Show me your ways, LORD, teach me your paths.

Psalms 25:4

19
Take Control

O Lord, my human nature tells me to take control,
to say things that curry favor,
to do things that ingratiate myself to others,
to make sure others know what I can do,
to protect myself, take care of myself,
promote myself, trust only myself.
O Lord, You are in control. You are the one I will trust.
You promote.
You watch over and protect your children.
The words I speak should only flow from your
love. O Lord, may your nature take over my
nature.
I surrender to you. Take control.

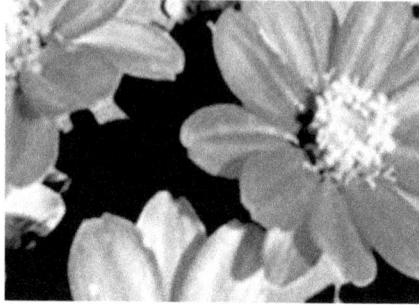

Is it not to share your food with
the hungry and to provide the
poor wanderer with shelter when
you see the naked, to clothe them,
and not to turn away from your
own flesh and blood?

Isaiah 58:7

20
Fasting

O Lord, teach me how to fast.

Not just the giving up of something, but the giving of

something. Not just a spiritual exercise of worship to know you

better, and gather to myself some great spiritual prowess.

But living out your love and purpose.

To change a life - not just the soul's destination.

Teach me, Lord, teach me.

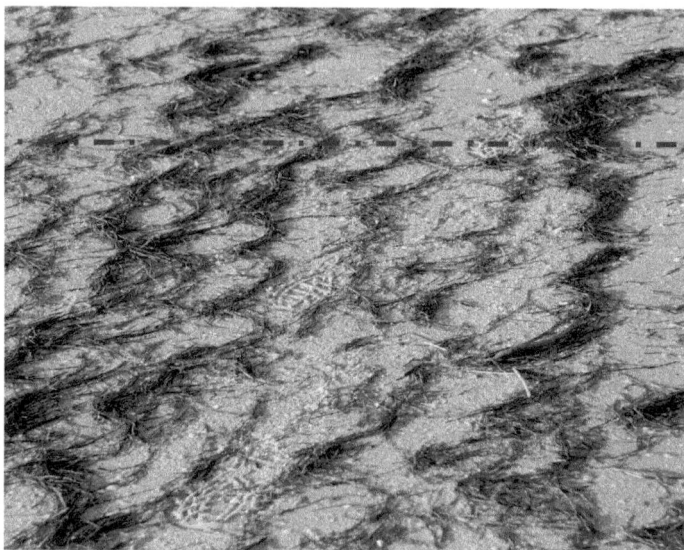

Your word, LORD, is eternal; it stands firm in the heavens.

Psalms 119:89

21
Your Word

O Lord, let me learn in silence; Let me hear your word,

May you speak the living word. Change my mind, change my heart.

Renew me, restore me, remind me.

Steel my will to walk in obedience.

May my heart be at peace in following your word.

Let my mind grasp the power of your word.

Your word brings life to my being.

Without your word there is only existence.

Speak and I will listen. Lead and I will follow. Rest and I will be still.

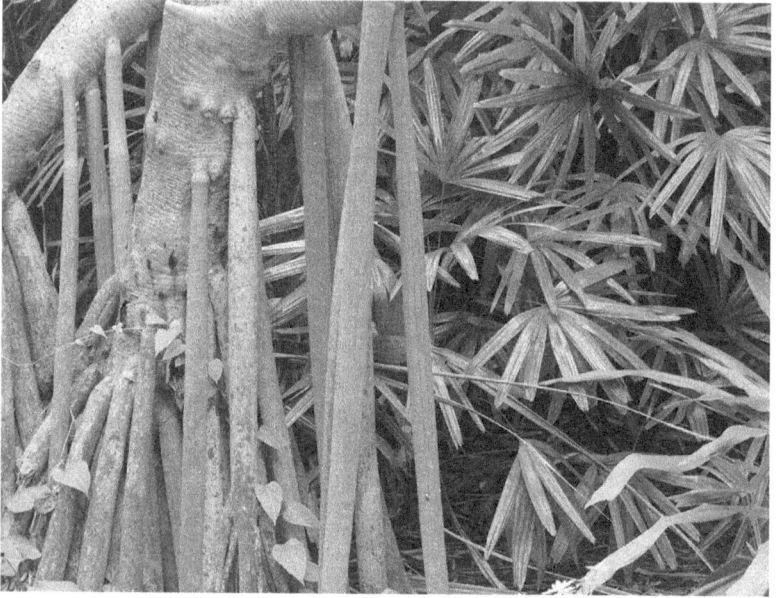

I called on your name, O LORD,
from the depths of the pit;
you heard my plea ...

Lamentations 3:55,56

22
Buried Alive

Lord, I have been buried alive,
Selfishness, self-doubt, self-pity
Self-absorption, and self-centeredness
Have buried me alive.
I am dead.
But You are my resurrection.
You are my Life.
Breathe into me your breath.

And I will live.

Selflessness because You are my provision.
Self-assurance because You are my strength.
Others-centered because You care for me.
You are the drink to quench my thirst
You are the food to feed my soul.

I live.

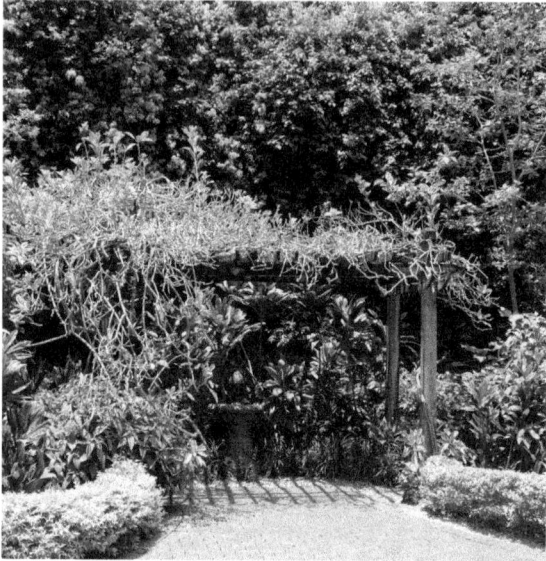

BE STILL before the LORD and wait patiently for him ...

Psalms 37:7

23
Waiting

Jesus, it is difficult to wait.
I'm not built for waiting.
Spontaneous, impetuous best describe me.
Teach me to wait.

I would sit at your feet.
I would wait in your presence.
I would listen for your words.
Help me know your voice.

Help me recognize Your whisper.
May I joy in Your laughter.
May I be silent in your discipline.
May I grasp Your words of life.

Your words are strength for the day.
Your touch is courage for the moment.
Your presence is protection from the circumstance.
Your silence is the power of friendship.

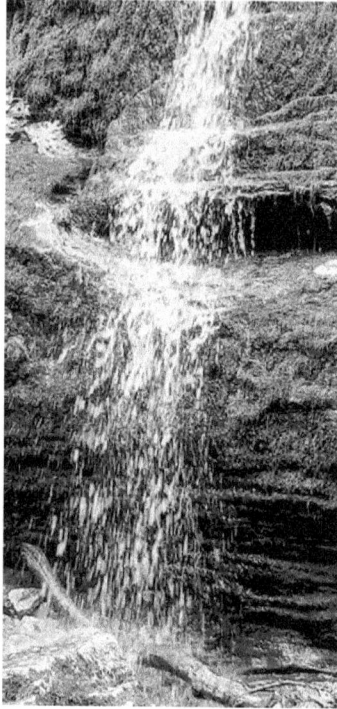

Sow righteousness for yourselves,
reap the fruit of unfailing love,
and break up your unplowed
ground; for it is time to seek
the LORD, until he comes and
showers his righteousness on you.

Hosea 10:12

24

Rain

O Lord, soak me in your heavenly rain.

Let every fiber of my being be drenched in Your love and mercy. Let

the power of Your presence satisfy my soul like the morning dew.

Wash me in your cleansing stream.

May my sin be wiped away like a flood in the desert.

May my thirst be satisfied by Your living water.

My You sooth my troubled soul with Your healing fountain.

May You overwhelm me like a waterfall.

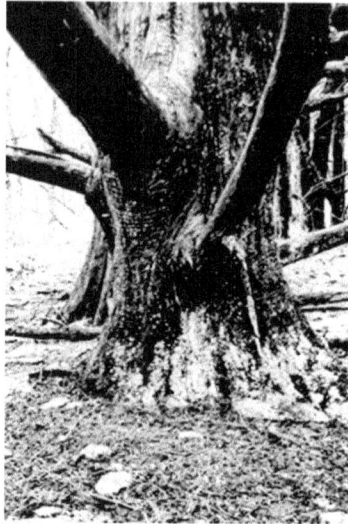

There is no one like you, LORD,
and there is no God but you,
as we have heard with
our own ears.

1 Chronicles 17:20

25
No One Like You

O Lord, there is no one like You.
You speak and the heavens fall into place,
Each word You speak is life itself.

There are no other gods.
My puny mind cannot grasp all You are,
But I know You are real.

May your Spirit take my spirit captive.
May He rule my body, mind, and soul.
I submit control!

Lead me in the right path.
Guide my steps.
I will follow you on this journey.

Help me grow in relationship with you.
Help me move from a babe in arms,
To brother and friend.

You call us to Yourself.
The Creator who walks with his creation.
There is no one like You.

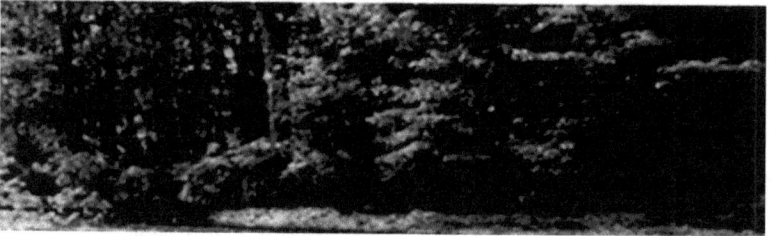

Remember, LORD, your great
mercy and love, for they are
from of old.

Psalms 25:6

26
Forgive Me

Jesus, forgive me for saying you don't care.
When things are not to my liking,
Or go contrary to my plans.

Forgive me for beating myself up,
When I make mistakes,
Or think I have failed.

Forgive me for those moments
I act like God,
Like I have all power.

Forgive me for accusing you of abandonment.
You cannot walk away,
You are my Savior, Brother, and Father.

Forgive me for acting like a child,
Throwing a tantrum,
When I don't get what I want.

Thank you for your forgiveness.
Thank you for your love.
Thank you for your life.

Do not worship any other god, for the LORD, whose name is Jealous, is a jealous God.

Exodus 34:14

27
Forgive Us

Jesus, forgive us for worshiping our acts of worship.

Forgive us for consuming the sacrifice we are bringing to you. Forgive us for bowing to the idol of success.

Forgive us for idolizing charismatic leaders who have no character.

Forgive us for serving self rather than others.

Forgive us for our lack of accountable relationships.

Forgive us for acting as if others do not count in our salvation journey.

Forgive us for remaining in the boxes of rules instead of the freedom of relationships.

Forgive us for living in legalism and license instead of love.

Forgive us for making lifestyle choices the litmus test for being part of the Family.

Forgive us for preaching grace and mercy and living judgment and criticism.

Forgive us Lord, Forgive us ...

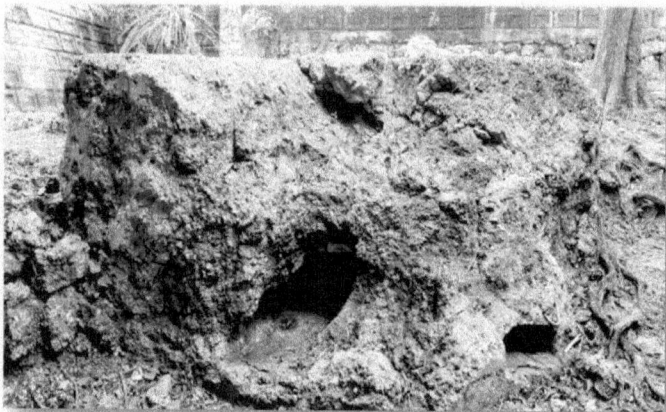

Test me, LORD, and try me,
examine my heart and my mind;
for I have always been mindful of
your unfailing love and have lived
in reliance on your faithfulness.

Psalms 26:2-3

28
Test Me

Jesus, when you test me in the furnace of affliction,
May the impurities all be burned away.

Make me as pure as silver and gold.

When I am in the flames of testing.

As steel is hardened in the furnace,
May my life become so resilient.

May I accept the fire as refining and not torture,
As discipline and not punishment,
As freedom and not imprisonment.

May I always remember,
Your Spirit is there in the midst of the Heat,
So ... I accept and submit to your refining.

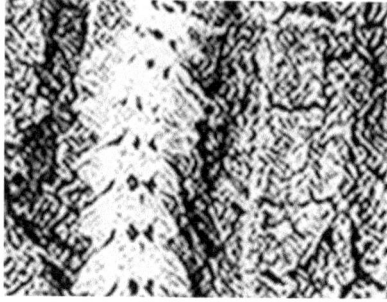

And we all, who with unveiled
faces contemplate the Lord's glory, are
being transformed into his
image with ever-increasing glory, which
comes from the Lord,
who is the Spirit.

2 Corinthians 3:18

29
Transformation

Jesus, transform me!
Show me what I am in You.
Cause my mind and heart to align with You.
Let my conforming be to you, not the world.

Show me what it is to live in Your Kingdom.
Help me see Your Reality not my reality.
Let my life reflect Your values.
Let my worship be 24/7, not an hour on Sundays.

Help me live in each moment.
Not the last one or the next one.
And in that moment live completely in you.
Jesus, transform me.

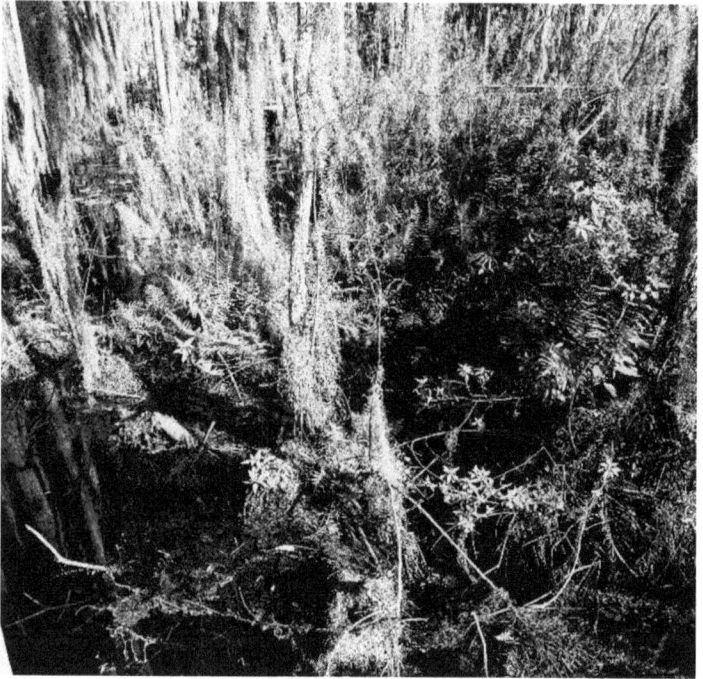

For it is commendable if someone bears up under the pain of unjust suffering because they are conscious of God.

1 Peter 2:19

30
Circumstantial Evidence

Jesus, help me understand
The path of least resistance.
It may not be the right way.

When things are going well,
And all doors fly open, You
may not be there.

Help me see that opposition,
And difficult situations may
not be suffering for you.

When oppression comes and
everything is contrary, It may
not be your discipline.

Show me that circumstance,
Good or bad
Are always on the path.

My faith and trust
are in you my Friend,
Not circumstantial evidence.

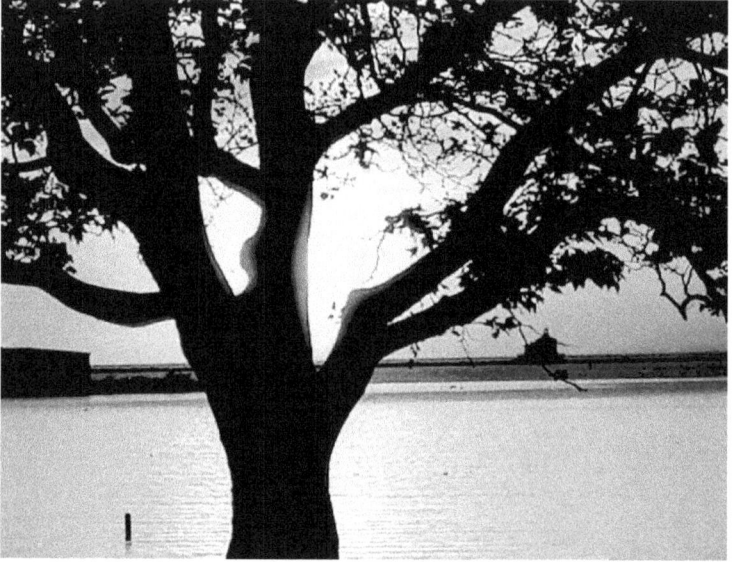

... fix your thoughts on Jesus.

Hebrews 3:1

31
Son Glasses

Jesus, my perspective is myopic and short sighted.
I can only see this moment.
And fantasize about the future.

Give me eyes to see,
What you want me to see.
Help me focus on You not the future.

Heal my blindness.
Give me sight.
Give me clarity.

No more rose-colored glasses.
No more bifocals.
No more contacts.

Change my prescription.
Help me focus on you.
Give me Son glasses.

... the Spirit who gives life has set you free from the law of sin and death.

Romans 8:2

32
Set Me Free

O Lord, set me free,
Free from the inglorious.
Free from the inconsequential. Free
from inconsistent.

Free from selfishness.
Free from self-assurance.
Free from self-centeredness.

Set me free from all that distracts,
Set me free from all that detracts,
Set me free from all that defeats.

Set me free to be an encourager, Set
me free to be a promoter,
Set me free to be a motivator.

Set me free for Your purpose.
Set me free to follow Your passions.
Set me free, Your life to practice .

Set me free to sacrifice for You.
Set me free to suffer for You.
Set me free to be sustained by You.

Set me free to walk in Your Way.
Set me free to grow in Your Word.
Set me free to live in Worship.

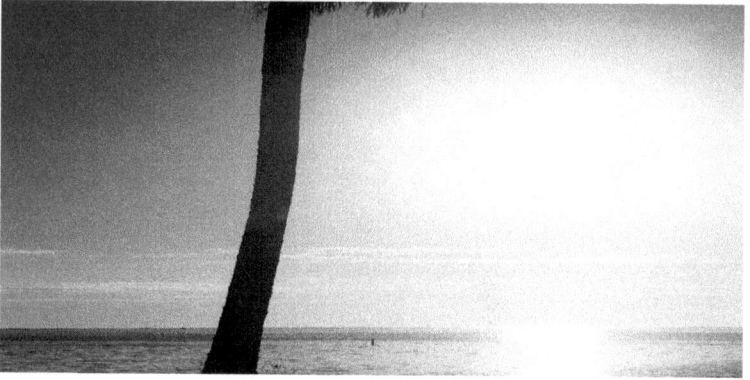

All of us, then, who are
mature should take such a
view of things.

Philippians 3:15

33
Kid No More

Jesus, I don' want to be a kid anymore!
I know I will always be a child, before the Father;
But I want to grow up, I want to keep growing up.

You say you are my brother.
Jesus, I want to be your brother.
I want to live like your brother.

Thank you for Your patience with me.
Thank you for Your mercy on me.
Thank you for sticking up for me.

Help me be an adult.
A mature member of the family.
Help me be prepared for eternity.

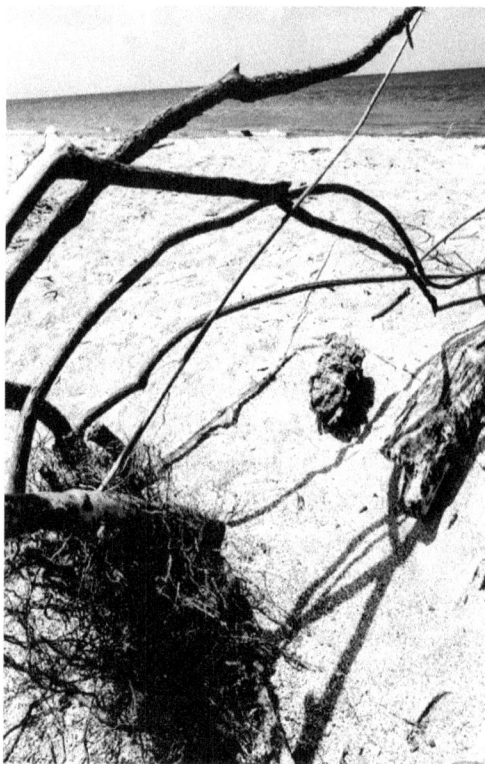

The LORD is close to the
brokenhearted and saves those
who are crushed in spirit.

Psalms 34:18

34
Sickness and Death

O Lord,
I know You are good.
I know You are loving.
I know You watch over us.
I know ...

Hear my prayer.
My heart is broken.
My mind is numb.
My body is in pain.

This path of sickness and death;
It is unfamiliar.
I don't want to be here.
I want off this path.
I submit to Your mercy.
I sleep in Your grace.
I will rest in Your goodness.
I Will believe ...

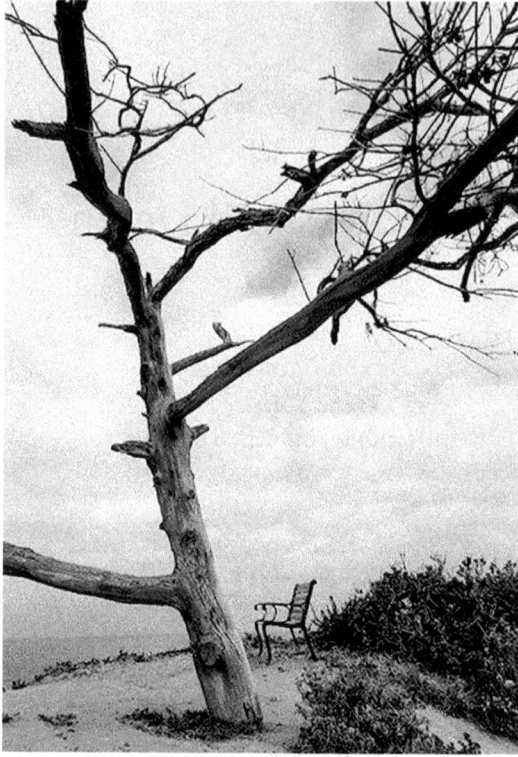

Test me, LORD, and try me,
examine my heart and my mind;
for I have always been mindful of
your unfailing love and have lived
in reliance on your faithfulness.

Psalms 26:2-3

35
Character

Jesus,
I know the most important thing is
not my comfort,
is not my career,
but my character.

Test me that I may be proven.
Protect me so that I may not fall.
Keep me from the pit of destruction.

Prove me.
Let the fire come.
Burn the dross away.

May all who see - rejoice.
May all who watch - glorify You.
May all who wonder - be convinced.

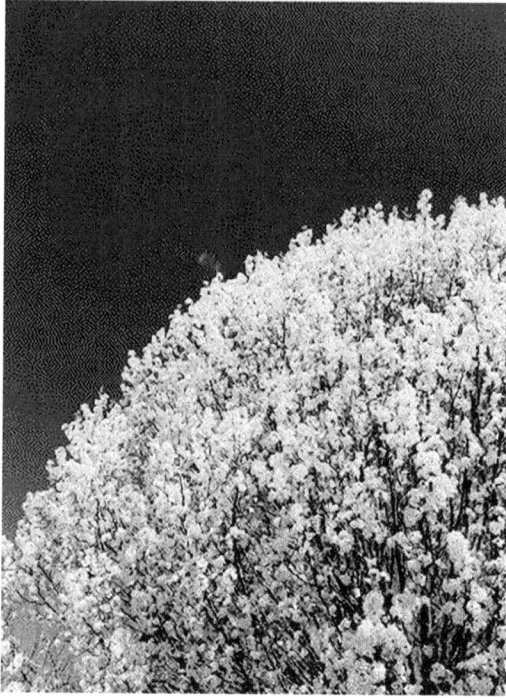

I press on toward the goal to win the prize for which God has called me heavenward in Christ Jesus.

Philippeans 3:14

36
Life Happens

O Lord,
I know life happens.

It is not punishment from You.

It is not the enemy winning.

Help me not to blame.

Help me not to accuse.

Help me not curse the circumstance.

I will trust You in the now.

I will have faith for the future.

I will not live in the past.

> *You   are   my   Provider.*
> *You are   my   Protector.*
> *You   are   my   Prosperity.*

Show me, LORD, my life's end
and the number of my days;
let me know
how fleeting my life is.

Psalms 39:4

37
Eternity

O Lord, help me focus on Eternity,
Not the things of this world;
Help me shake off this earthly entrapment.

Let me live in each moment.

Let me count the number of my days.

Let each action, each word have eternal value.

Change my heart to live with an eternal perspective.
Not the getting and the keeping,
And the getting more.

Help me to live out Kingdom values not earthly values.

Let the getting be for giving.

Let the having be for sharing.

Let Who has me be more important that what I have.

Let Eternity say, "He lived well."

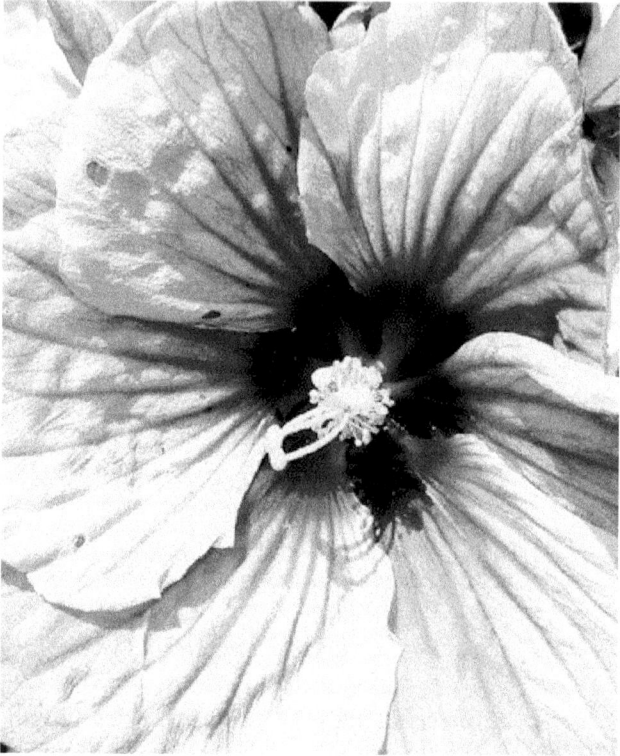

"Father, if you are willing, take this cup from me; yet not my will, but yours be done."

Luke 22:42

38
Not My Will

Even when circumstance goes in contrary direction.

You are at work;
Teaching us, guiding us, growing us, molding us, refining us.

You are perfecting us;
If we allow you to take us through the circumstance.

Let me learn not to feel betrayed by circumstance,
or fight against it,
or finally desert it.

Help me understand why circumstance is there:
Fulfilling Your work, Your plan for my life.

As Jesus prayed ...
Not my will but Yours be done.

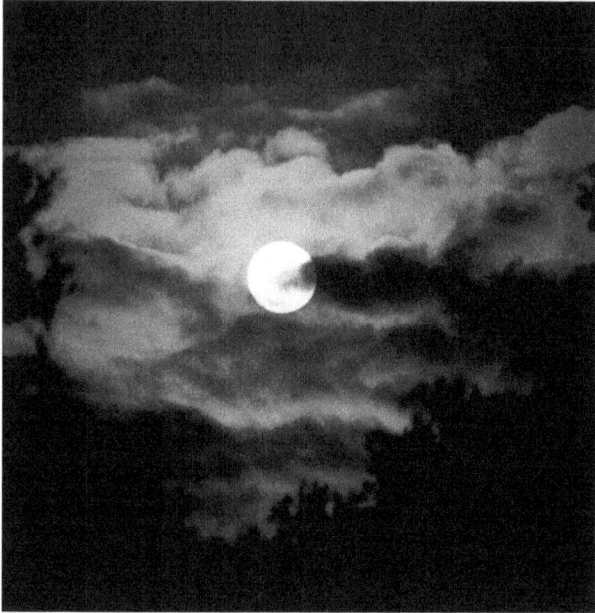

Give careful thought to the
paths for your feet
and be steadfast in all
your ways.

Proverbs 4:26

39
Following You

O Lord, Keep me on the path of your choosing.
I am easily distracted by others.
New challenges constantly call my name.
Circumstances demand attention.
Help me keep my eyes on You.

Let my feet follow You,
regardless of the surroundings,
regardless of the voices screaming,
regardless of the enticing songs.
Your path is true, it is secure, it does not wonder.

O Lord, your Spirit is my guide,
My Comforter, my Friend, my Protector.
I choose your path,
Even when I cannot see around the bend
Or over the rise.
Even when it looks like a dead-end.

I will trust You, I will rejoice in You.
You cannot lead me astray.
I will praise your name.

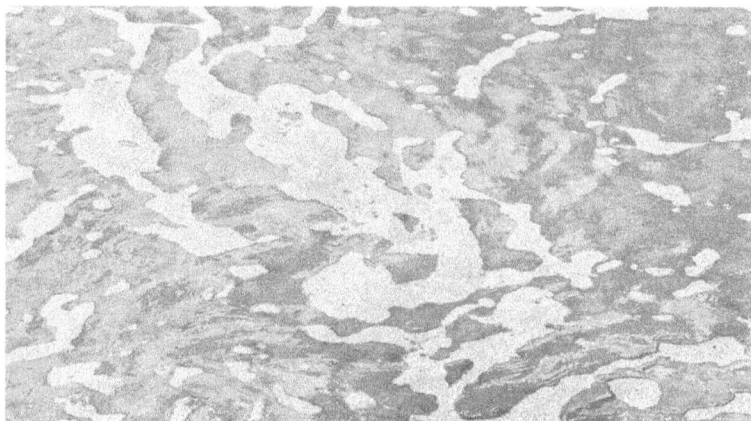

Then the LORD spoke to Job
out of the storm.

Psalms 26:2-3

40
The Storm Still Rages

O Lord, The storm still rages.
But I am safe in you.
My enemies have plotted against me.
But you know their plans.

Destruction comes to claim his prize.
But you laugh in his face.
Confusion comes to spread his lies.
But your truth intervenes.
Frustration taunts me.
But your peace fills my soul.
Depression's darkness tries to overwhelm.
But your light explodes all around me.
Temptation arrives with ugly purpose.
But you answer the door.

You are my God.
In You I will be.

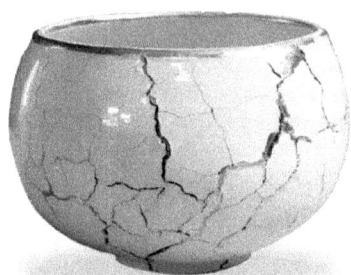

Printed in the USA
CPSIA information can be obtained
at www.ICGtesting.com
JSHW010543010823
45655JS00002B/75

9 798218 227395